Heal Your Gut

The Ultimate Beginner's Heal Your Leaky Gut Diet Guide - Finally Heal & Restore Balance In Your Body

(+50 Nourishing & Repairing Recipes)

By Jennifer Louissa

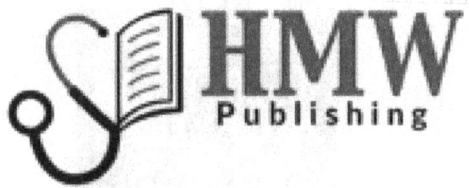

For more great books visit:

HMWPublishing.com

Get another book for Free

I want to thank you for purchasing this book and offer you another book (just as long and valuable as this book), "Health & Fitness Mistakes You Don't Know You're Making", completely free.

Visit the link below to signup and receive it:

www.hmwpublishing.com/gift

In this book, I will break down the most common health & fitness mistakes, you are probably committing right now, and I will reveal how you can easily get in the best shape of your life!

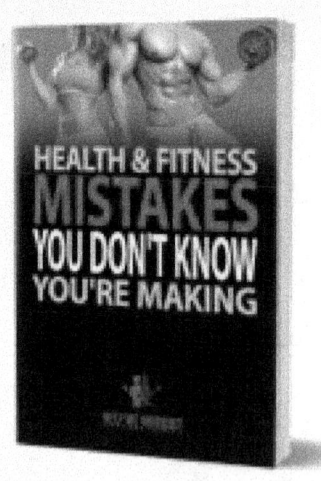

In addition to this valuable gift, you will also have an opportunity to get our new books for free, enter giveaways, and receive other valuable emails from me. Again, visit the link to sign up:

www.hmwpublishing.com/gift

TABLE OF CONTENTS

Introduction 1

Chapter 1: Your Gut and Its Significance to Your Health 4

Understanding the Human Anatomy 5
The Body is a Human Host 5
What Determines your Gut Health? 6
The Gut Barrier 8

Gut: The Second Brain 10

The Gut: The Key To Your Immune System
.... 12

Chapter 2: Causes and Effects of Poor Gut and .. 14

Flora Imbalance 14

Common Leading Causes of Poor Gut Health
.... 14
Chronic Stress 14
Dysbiosis 15
Environmental Contaminants 16
Overconsumption of Alcoholic Beverages 17
Poor Food Choices 17
Use of Medications 18
Food and Environmental Sensitivities 18
Lectins 19

Effects of Flora Imbalance 20
Autoimmune Illnesses 20
Mental Health 21
Poor Immune Health 22

Link to Type 2 Diabetes 24
Small Intestinal Bacterial Overgrowth (SIBO) 26
Chapter 3: Spot Signs of a Leaky Gut 27

Symptoms in the Gut 27

General Symptoms 28
Leaky Gut Without Symptoms 31

Chapter 4: Heal Your Unhealthy Gut 32

How to Maintain and Restore a Healthy Gut
....32

Eat Traditional Foods 34
Consume Lactic Acid Yeast Wafers 35
Consider Intermittent Fasting 37
Practice Meditation 37
Do Some Exercise 38
Take High-Quality Probiotics 38
Doing a Leaky Test 39
Treat Intestinal Pathogens 39
Consider Including Whole Foods in your Diet 40

Chapter 5: Bounce Back to Life with Gut-Healthy Recipes 45

The Bone Broth and Other Soup Recipes .45

Recipe #1 - Bone Broth 45
Recipe #2 - Chicken Zoodle Bone Broth Soup 48
Recipe #3 - Herb Roasted Bone Marrow 51
Recipe #4 - Homemade Beef Broth 53
Recipe #5 - Thai Carrot Soup 56
Recipe #6 - Mussels Soup 58
Recipe #7 - Creamy Potato and Chicken Soup 60

Recipe #8 - Chicken Zoodle Faux Pho............64
Recipe #9 - Crock Pot Pho............................66
Recipe #10 - Creamy Broccoli Soup 70

Detoxifying Smoothies, Juices, and Other Drinks 72

Recipe #11- Natural Ginger Ale 72
Recipe #12- Coconut Water Kefir....................74
Recipe #13 - Orange Juice Detox.....................76
Recipe #14 - Gut-Soothing Ginger & Slippery Elm Tea 78
Recipe #15 - Gut-Healing Smoothie.................80
Recipe #16 - Anti-Inflammatory Turmeric Milk 82
Recipe #17 - Cilantro - Cucumber Juice..........84
Recipe #18 - Cucumber Mint Drink 85
Recipe #19 - Revitalizing Papaya Smoothie....86
Recipe #20 - Go Green Gut Recipe..................87

Anti-Leak Food Recipes for the Gut 89

Recipe #21- Superfood for Gut Burger............89
Recipe #22 - Herb-Crusted Salmon 91
Recipe #23 - Gut-Friendly Breakfast Scramble 94
Recipe #24 - Coconut Chicken Curry 96
Recipe #25 - Bacon-Packed Potatoes 99
Recipe#26 - Meaty Zucchini with Onions and Mushrooms...102
Recipe #27 - Turkey Tortilla Sandwich 104
Recipe #28- Cucumber and Crab Salad 106
Recipe #29 - Simple Broccoli Salad.................108

Recipe #30 - Israeli Salad with Grilled Chicken 110
Recipe #31 - Lemony Omelet with Smoked Trout 112
Recipe #32 - Zucchini Noodles..........................114
Recipe #33 - Healthy Gut Zesty Salad with Fish Cakes..........................116
Recipe #34 - Bacon, Chicken and Pecan Salad 119
Recipe #35 - Spanish Sausage and Baked Eggs 121
Recipe #36 - Italian-Style Pan-Fried Broccoli 124
Recipe #37 - Smoked Salmon Breakfast Delight 126
Recipe #38 - Spicy Shrimp-Avocado Turret...129
Recipe #39 - Baked Sea Bass with Lemon Caper Dressing..........................132
Recipe #40 - Bacon Omelet Wedges - Summer Salad Recipe 135
Recipe #41 - Salmon and Spinach With Tartare Cream..........................138
Recipe #42 - Quick and Easy Black Rice Mix..140
Recipe #43 - Oat Porridge with Fruit Delight.142
Recipe #44 - Coconut Chicken with Spinach ..144
Recipe #45 - Stir-Fried Gingered Salmon........146
Recipe #46 - The Ultimate Healthy Gut Noodles 148
Recipe #47 - Kombucha..........................150
Recipe #48 - Crunchy Egg Roll..........................152
Recipe #49 - Daikon-Endive Salad..................156

Recipe #50 - Zucchini Pasta with Sausage and
    Roasted Garlic Sauce...................................160
Final Words..162
About the Co-Author...163

Introduction

I want to thank you and congratulate you for purchasing the "The Ultimate Beginner's Guide To Healing Your Gut" book.

Living in this modern era entails many consequences including issues with stress, anxiety, and depression. However, you may not realize that all these are clear indicators of problems linking to your gut health. Though you may find it surprising to know that the bacteria in your gut can impact many parts of your body, including your mental health, it is exactly what studies are telling us now.

Intestinal permeability or leaky gut is hard to diagnose with symptoms that are somehow similar to many diseases, but one of its major causes is the overgrowth of candida, which comprises the intestinal structure.

This book, "Heal Your Gut: The Ultimate Beginner's Guide To Healing a Leaky Gut" contains proven steps and effective strategies on how you can heal your gut and save yourself from chronic and deadly diseases. You will likewise discover how you can enjoy savory and sumptuous delicious meals while helping your gut recover from an imbalanced gut flora.

Moreover, you will learn why a healthy eating lifestyle is essential in maintaining a healthy gut. Likewise, you will how to protect yourself from the attack of harmful microbes, which can cause your immune system to break down and leave yourself defenceless. Lastly, a sample gut-friendly plan and anti-leaky gut recipes are included to make your meals complete, filling, and enjoyable! Thanks again for purchasing this book, I hope you enjoy reading it!

Also, before you get started, I recommend you **joining our email newsletter** to receive updates on any upcoming new book releases or promotions. You can sign-up for free, and as a bonus, you will receive a free gift. Our "*Health & Fitness Mistakes You Don't Know You're Making*" book! This book has been written to demystify, expose the top do's and don'ts and to finally equip you with the information you need to get in the best shape of your life. Due to the overwhelming amount of mis-information and lies told by magazines and self-proclaimed "gurus", it's becoming harder and harder to get reliable information to get in shape. As opposed to having to go through dozens of biased, unreliable and untrustworthy sources to get your health & fitness information. Everything you need to help you has been broken down in this book for you to easily follow and to immediately get results to achieve your desired fitness goals in the shortest amount of time.

Once again, to join our free email newsletter and to receive a free copy of this valuable book, please visit the link and signup now: www.hmwpublishing.com/gift

Chapter 1: Your Gut and Its Significance to Your Health

Many centuries ago, it was Hippocrates who said that diseases begins in the gut, but it was only these past two decades that research studies had proven and disclosed how right he was when he said this. Studies revealed that our gut indeed is crucial to our overall health and that an unhealthy gut is a perfect host to a wide range of diseases. This includes obesity, arthritis, depression, chronic fatigue, inflammatory diseases, and much more.

This discovery leads many researchers to believe that taking care of intestinal health and restoring back the efficient function and integrity of the gut barrier will be the major concern of the medical word in the 21st century.

Understanding the Human Anatomy

Imagine a computer system made up of various parts that functions separately and yet works together to make the whole computer system be functional. Thus, when one part of it becomes nonfunctional, it affects the entire process and ultimately leads to its total breakdown, if not repaired on time.

Our human body functions exactly as a computer does. It is made up of different systems that are somehow interrelated and together work towards giving us a healthy physical body. So when there is problem with one part - like our digestive system, it affects our overall health. And if we neglect or refuse to give it proper care or attention, it will lead to a more serious problem in the long run.

The Body is a Human Host

Our body is a host to billions of germs, viruses, bacteria fungi, and other microbial agents - in fact, our body is a microbiota. A human microbiota is made up of 10-100 trillion symbiotic microbiota. Luckily for us that most of these are beneficial to our health. The majority of these little creatures we are carrying in our body reside in the gut weighing approximately 1.5 kilograms and of a thousand different species. Many of these species are yet to be discovered by science.

Vital to our gut biome is the multiple strains of Bifidobacterium that inhabit the large intestine and the lactobacillus that inhabits the small intestines. Through various factors like stress, poor diet, and use of antibiotics can make a change in their ratio and location in the intestines which can result in a multitude of health issues.

What Determines your Gut Health?

There are two significant and various interrelated variables which determine your gut health: the gut flora or intestinal microbiota and the gut barrier.

A human gut contains a considerable number of bacteria that is 10 times more than the quantity of human cells in the entire body with 400 known diverse species of bacteria. Your gut flora or intestinal flora is a community of microorganisms occupying your digestive tract. They constitute a part of the human microbiota which is comprised of all organisms dwelling within your body and helps inhibit the growth of harmful bacteria causing infections.

It was only recently that humankind was able to understand the extent of the role of gut flora in human health and diseases. Included in the functions of the gut flora which are vital to the human life are the following:

- Promote normal gastrointestinal functions

- Protects from infection

- Regulates metabolism

- Comprises more than 75 percent of our immune system

A dysregulated gut flora has been associated with diseases ranging from depression, autism and other autoimmune conditions like hashimoto's, type 1 diabetes, and inflammatory bowel disease.

The Gut Barrier

Now, we know that our gut serves as a shelter to these numerous bacteria, but have you ever considered what will happen if these gut contents are scattered out of it?

The gut is a hollow tube that passes through the mouth and ends at the anus. Anything that comes in the mouth and isn't digested and broken down into nutrients will move right out to the other end of the passage. The gut barrier primary function is to decide what gets in and what stays out of the body. It serves as the body's gatekeeper.

Hence, when there's a leak in the intestinal barrier as it becomes permeable like in a leaky gut syndrome, large protein molecules can escape through the bloodstream. Since these molecules should remain inside the gut, their escape results to the body automatically mounting an immune response and attacks them. Studies show that such attacks pay a significant role in the development and onset of autoimmune disease. In fact, Dr. Alessio Fasano, an expert in mucosal biology believes that a leaky gut is a precondition to developing autoimmune diseases.

Likewise, there is growing evidence that an intestine leak pays a pathogenic role in different autoimmune diseases like celiac disease and type 1 diabetes. Therefore, it is necessary to strengthen the intestinal barrier to develop autoimmunity against various diseases. This also proves that the integrity of the gut barrier is crucial in the prevention of autoimmune diseases.

This discovery holds that the gut barrier mostly determines whether your body tolerates or reacts to refuse the toxic substances that you ingest from outside sources. The damage in the intestinal barrier, which is imminent in a leaky gut, caused by food toxins like gluten and chemical substances like arsenic or BPA can generate an immune response which affects not only the gut but other organs and tissues in the body. These include the kidney, liver. Pancreas, brain, and the whole skeletal system.

It's crucial to understand that you don't have to experience gut symptoms to have a leaky gut. A leaky gut can have other manifestations of skin problems including eczema, psoriasis, and autoimmune conditions which affect the thyroid or joints, mental illness depression, autism spectrum disorder, and much more.

Researchers have also discovered that a protein called zonulin can increase intestinal permeability in humans and animals. In most autoimmune diseases - multiple sclerosis, type 1 diabetes, celiac disease, rheumatoid arthritis, and inflammatory bowel disease, abnormally high levels of zonulin were found and are usually characterized by a leaky gut.

Gut: The Second Brain

Ever wondered why we experience stomach cramps or butterflies in our stomach when we have stage frights just as our mind seems to stop working? There are also times when we rely on our gut feeling to make decisions or trust our gut instinct to sense danger. We are often told to check in onour gut when we are faced with situations that test our nerves and determination. It is because we have two sets of the brain - with one encased in a skull and what we often referred to as our head. The other one is less popular, but likewise significant to our life and is found there inside our stomach - the gut.

These two brains are greatly interconnected and function almost in the same manner - sending signals to other parts of the body and alerting them when danger is coming. When one brain is upset, so is the other according to the science journalist, Sandra Blakeslee for New York Times.

The digestive tract contains over than a million nerve cells almost equal to that found in the spinal cord. There are more nerve cells found in the digestive system than in the peripheral nervous system. To top it all, vital neurotransmitters that are located in the brain including serotonin, glutamate, dopamine, nitric oxide, and norepinephrine are likewise found in large quantity in the gut. The body's natural opiates - Enkephalins are also found in the intestinal tract and so are benzodiazepines, a psychoactive chemical that controls the mood. Thus when you have a weak digestive health, it can lead to mood disorders and other forms of neurological disorders.

The Gut: The Key To Your Immune System

Aside from its significance to your mental and emotional health, the digestive system plays a crucial role in your natural immunity to various types of illnesses. It is because your gut is sterile, being an ecosystem of bacteria and yeast which are most beneficial to your health, though there are others that are toxic.

When the intestinal ecosystem is healthy, that beneficial yeast and bacteria can keep harmful microorganism at bay in your digestive tract. But when there is an imbalance or when dysbiosis occurs, this will result in an overgrowth of fungus and other pathogens leading to numerous gastrointestinal disorders.

Like all ecosystems, some chemical substance found in antibiotics, fluoride in water, preservative and additive in foods, stimulants in coffee and a lot of hard-to-digest foods such as improperly prepared whole grains can alter the delicate balance of the digestive tract. Once the balance in the quantity of microorganisms in your gut is out of balance, giving way to the proliferation of harmful bacteria, bad bacteria begin to produce toxins that can weaken the immune response. They can also interfere with the proper absorption of nutrients. It is why there are cases where a person can consume a nutrient-rich diet and remain deficient in appropriate nutrients because of an inadequate digestive system.

Chapter 2: Causes and Effects of Poor Gut and

Flora Imbalance

It's hard to pinpoint a single cause for a leaky gut syndrome, but some frequent contributors often lead to disturbing the flora balance in the gut. Let's discuss some of these factors that cause ill health to your gut.

Common Leading Causes of Poor Gut Health

Chronic Stress

When you are experiencing a prolonged stress, your immune system's ability to respond quickly is altered affecting your ability to heal. Every time your body feels that you are in an emergency situation and this is what happens when you are under stress, it prepares itself to be in a "fight or flight" mode and produces hormones like adrenaline to help you out of danger. However, when this often happens, there is overproduction in your adrenaline making your insulin-resistant as it goes on and on, your body loses its ability to sense danger. It can no longer tell the difference between the typical day to day stress and real stress.

Once in a real state of danger like being face to face with a vicious beast, the body reacts to such stressor by producing less secretory IgA or sIgA, one of the front lines of the body's immune defense system and lessens DHEA - an anti-aging, anti-stress adrenal hormone. It likewise slows down the digestion and peristalsis, decreases blood flow to digestive organs, and produces metabolites.

Dysbiosis

Dysbiosis is a condition wherein there is a microbial imbalance inside the body which contributes to the existence of a leaky gut. When there is an overproduction of candida, a fungus responsible for nutrient absorption and digestion when in contained comparable levels in the body, it can break down the walls of the intestine lining and penetrates into the bloodstream. Candidiasis must be taken into consideration when leaky gut is suspected. There are other parasites and microbes like salmonella, amoebas, shigella, Helicobacter, giardia, and many others that cause irritation to the intestinal lining and cause gastrointestinal symptoms. People with digestive illness or a history of it have a greater tendency to acquire leaky gut syndrome.

Environmental Contaminants

Every day, we are exposed to numerous environmental and household chemicals which put stress on our immune defenses and breaking the body's ability to self-repair. This can lead to a chronic delay of necessary routine repairs. Our immune system pays attention to many areas at one time and those far from the digestive system are affected - connective tissues are breaking down as the body loses trace minerals like calcium, magnesium, and potassium. Toxic chemicals deplete our reserves of buffering minerals, causing acidosis in the cells and tissue and swelling in the cells.

Overconsumption of Alcoholic Beverages

Although alcoholic drinks contain some nutrients, it takes many nutrients to metabolize. Among these are the B-complex vitamins. Alcoholic beverages contain substances that are also toxic to cells. When alcohol is metabolized in the liver, toxins are either broken down or further stored in the body. Alcohol abuse puts a strain on the liver and this affects digestive competency and further damages the intestinal tract.

Poor Food Choices

Consumption of low-fiber diet can increase the time of food digestion, allowing toxic by-products to accumulate and cause irritation in the gut mucosa. Diets of highly processed foods likewise injure the intestinal lining and they are invariably low in fiber and nutrients but contains a high level of food additives, restructured fats, and sugar. This kind of foods promotes inflammation of the Gastrointestinal (GI) tract. Therefore it is essential to know and remember that even foods that we thought of as healthful like wheat, eggs, and milk can, in fact, irritate the gut lining.

Use of Medications

There are medications such as nonsteroidal drugs like Advil, Motrin, and aspirin that can damage brush borders allowing partially digested food particles along with toxins and microbes to get into the bloodstream. Steroid drugs and birth control likewise create conditions that help feed fungi that damage the intestinal lining. Other things that can significantly disrupt the GI balance are chemotherapy medications and radiation.

Food and Environmental Sensitivities

Food, along with environmental sensitivities may be the cause of a leaky gut syndrome. These sensitivities, likewise referred to as delayed hypersensitivity differs from real food allergies. The widespread of these sensitivities is more widely-recognized today than in previous years as around 24 percent of American adults claimed that they have food and environmental sensitivities.

Lectins

Primarily found in legumes, lectins induce mast cells to produce histamine. The gut barrier in our intestine is meant to keep bacteria in our food away from getting into your bloodstream. Histamine, an inflammatory mediator-induced by mast cells which are part of the immune system are also found in the food that we consumed and these can compromise the gut barrier. They bind themselves to the intestinal mucosa to make it more leaky and porous causing the leaky gut.

Effects of Flora Imbalance

Autoimmune Illnesses

An autoimmune disease can occur when your body recognizes healthy cells as foreign objects resulting in inflammation and eventually leading to a total breakdown of your immune system. When your body immune system is trying to eradicate healthy cells, then this renders you helpless and without defense,

Although the exact cause of autoimmune diseases is unknown, it is speculated that they occur when there is an overgrowth of bad bacteria in the body. Currently, there are more than 80 known autoimmune diseases that are hard to recognize and are sharing similar symptoms. Some of these disorders include rheumatoid arthritis, Crohn's, and ulcerative colitis.

Mental Health

Within your intestinal wall are 500 million neurons that make up your enteric nervous system (ENS) which plays a vital role in producing around 30 different neurotransmitters. The ENS or the second brain as it is called is responsible for balancing your mood, keeping your overall mental health in check and reducing stress and anxiety. The collection of neurons in the ENS has created out the same cellular tissue like that of the brain and significantly influence your thoughts and feeling.

In various research studies using mice, researchers were able to establish the fact that you can completely change the behavior of the mice by changing their gut bacteria. In one experiment, a group of timid mice were given the gut bacteria taken from a group of mice who were brave and adventurous. As a result, the group of frightened mice was able to adapt to the behavior of the outgoing group of mice after the transfer of healthy gut bacteria. This research study proved that your gut affects your brain. Hence, if you are struggling with brain fog, anxiety, stress, depression or mental fatigue, then it is time for you to clean your gut!

Poor Immune Health

It is a fact that about 75 percent of the immune system is found in your Gastrointestinal (GI) tract. It is because your microbiome creates a significant impact on the digestive process and numerous issues can literally disable this self-healing mechanism and prevent it from performing to its maximum potential.

The Leaky Gut Syndrome as an example is a condition wherein your gut or intestinal lining or wall becomes permeable permitting toxins to leak out and be carried throughout your body through the bloodstream where it combines. When this happens, this is serious as your immune system recognizes it as foreign invaders and attacks them. Though at first, this is helpful to your body unless the leak or holes in your gut are fixed, this condition will continue and eventually deteriorate your immune system as it works around the clock trying to search and attack those foreign invaders. This severely weakened state of your immune system is sure to leave you susceptible to all sorts of infections and viruses as your body cannot defend itself. Here are some illnesses that can result from a weak and unhealthy immune system.

- Asthma and Allergies
- Antibiotic Associated Diarrhea
- Autoimmune Disease
- Cancer
- Dental Cavities
- Depression and Anxiety
- Autism
- Eczema, Psoriasis, and Dermatitis
- Eczema, Psoriasis, and Dermatitis
- Gastric Ulcers

- Obesity

- Malnutrition

- Diabetes

- Inflammatory Bowel Disease

The bottom line here is that when your digestive system is compromised, it also puts a strain and weakens your immune system. When your body is healthy, your immune system is active and effective in defending you against sickness. But when you are constantly with nagging coughs, sore throats, and colds, then you are most likely to have a leaky gut. Therefore, focus on it and heal your leaky gut before it totally vanquishes your immune system.

Link to Type 2 Diabetes

Recent studies discovered that there is a direct link between type 2 diabetes and an unhealthy gut. The study indicated that people with type 2 diabetes had high levels of bad bacteria that are damaging to gut health. Dr, Mark Hyman had somehow established the fact that obesity and diabetes are closely related. He further pointed out that once a person is obese, there is always a big chance that he has diabetes or in a pre-diabetic stage and this possibility exponentially increases with weight gained.

It is crucial to understand the connection between weight and diabetes. Many case studies has proven that a less diverse microbiome leads to weight gain and obesity. Recent statistics reported that 75 percent of the Americans are overweight and 20 percent of them are labeled as obese. With this rise in statistics, diabetes is almost becoming an epidemic. However, following a clean and healthy lifestyle can help you establish a diverse and robust microbiome that your body needs to remain healthy and prevent acquiring this death-leading illness.

Small Intestinal Bacterial Overgrowth (SIBO)

Small Intestinal Bacterial Overgrowth is the malfunction of the small intestine due to excessive growth of bacteria. Once these bacteria interact with food nutrients and food particles, it leads to a fermentation which can result in a wide range of symptoms.

Researchers suspect that the combination of decreased pancreatic enzymes, gut motility, and bile acids cause the onset of SIBO. Risk of SIBO is significantly affected by several factors that are often related to reduced functions and efficiency of the intestines. If left unattended for long, SIBO can a deficiency in nutrients -vitamins and minerals. Symptoms include digestive stress and severe nutrient deficiency.

Chapter 3: Spot Signs of a Leaky Gut

Your intestines are the portal to good health. When you have a healthy gut, there is a significant percentage that your overall state of health is most likely to be at its best. However, a weakened state of your gut is an indicator that something is wrong with your body and if not diagnosed earlier, can create havoc not only to your digestive system but can have a damaging effect on other systems in your physical body. So to spot signs of a leaky gut, there are some of the symptoms you need to be aware of.

Symptoms in the Gut

Some symptoms are concentrated in the gut.

- Bloating

- Ongoing diarrhea

- Gas

- Candida overgrowth

- Constipation

Symptoms can be detected throughout the body and still be attributed to factors that have something to do with your lifestyle. Inflammation can cause the gap in the intestinal lining to widen. Every time your immune systems detects the presence of particles that escape through the bloodstream, regardless of whether these are harmful or not, the defensive cells attack even healthy cells creating inflammation in the body.

General Symptoms

General signs of the gut disorder include:

- Food allergies

- Chronic fatigue

- Arthritis

- Joint pains

- General/seasonal allergies

- Skin rashes related to inflammation

- Weakened Immune System from overexertion

- Nutritional Deficiencies

- Brain-Related Symptoms

The digestive tract is said to contain the second highest number of nerves and communicates with the brain. This is according to a research study about the Emerging role of a gut-brain relationship conducted by Jocelyn J. and Kasper L.H. of Dartmouth College in New Hampshire (2014).

Symptoms related to the brain include:

- Moods

- Anxiety

- Depression

- Brain fog

More severe conditions arising from the leaky gut are also signs of its presence.

- Lupus
- Diabetes
- Hashimoto
- Rheumatoid Arthritis
- Celia
- IBS
- Crohn's
- Neurological Symptoms
- Alzheimer's disease
- General anxiety
- Headache/migraine
- Autism spectrum

- Fibromyalgià

- Multiple Sclerosis

- Neuropathy

Leaky Gut Without Symptoms

Increased permeability in the intestine and small points of inflammation often don't show anybody's signs and are not usually cause for concern. However numerous gaps in the intestines are accompanied by symptoms including:

- Bloating

- Cramping

- Gas

- Chronic fatigue which worsens after meals.

Chapter 4: Heal Your Unhealthy Gut

In maintaining a healthy gut, the first important thing you need to consider is to avoid all those elements stated in the previous chapters that are inimical to the gut flora and damage the intestinal barrier. Though of course, there are some instances when we can't control this like in cases of chronic stress and infections or when our lineage carries defective genes. However, even if you are already exposed to some of these harmful factors, still there are some ways to restore your gut flora.

How to Maintain and Restore a Healthy Gut

Here are some ways to consider in maintaining and restoring a healthy gut. When thinking about the restoration of our bio flora and gut bacteria, the first things we think of are the probiotic foods and supplements. Probiotics are the term used in the nutritional world to call bacteria that we intentionally eat for health benefits. They function in opposite to how antibiotics work in our body. However, they are just part of the many things we need to consider. You could fill up your body with probiotics but if you continue living on unhealthy lifestyle - including habits that will keep damaging your gut bacteria such as drinking highly chlorinated water and taking antibiotics, sure enough, you will just end up creating more damage to your intestinal lining.

Remember that for the beneficial microorganisms to survive, grow, and flourish, they need a stable ecosystem. An ideal pH level must be 7 and lower than that means more acidity. A much higher level over 7 means more alkaline. Since your colon needs to be slightly acidic to inhibit the growth of undesirable bacteria including Shigella, Salmonella, and E.coli. the ideal pH level must be between 6.7-6.9. For those who have no idea of what a pH level is all about, pH level refers to the level of alkalinity or acidity of water-soluble substances.

The best way, therefore to restore the number of good bacteria is to increase the acidity level particularly in your gut to promote the growth of Lactobacillus bacteria or "useful bacteria." These type of bacteria are well known for their beneficial effects to your gut. To accomplish this purpose, here are some proven and effective ways to do it. By merely observing these ways, you can help improve the condition of your gut barrier and flora.

Eat Traditional Foods

Eating regularly foods that contain a lot of friendly probiotic bacteria like those found in traditional fermented foods can enhance and improve the gut flora. These foods are rich in beneficial lactic-producing bacteria which naturally turn milk products sour and caused vegetables to ferment.

When talking about foods that undergo fermentation process, your options aren't limited to fermented soy or sauerkraut. Other fantastic options are considered "fermented," including tea, yogurt, and various vegetables. Here are 9 fermented foods you should include in your gut.

- Yogurt
- Natto
- Kefir
- Kombucha
- Kimchi
- Tempeh
- Pickles
- Lassi

Consume Lactic Acid Yeast Wafers

Consuming traditional foods or taking probiotic supplements are often enough for some people to increase the number of beneficial bacteria in the gut. But some individuals require an additional step to be able to restore the intestinal flora. Lactic acid yeast wafers can provide you with the same result you can get from consuming traditional fermented foods or probiotic supplements by restoring the flora of the lower bowel.

Lactic Acid Yeast is just a modified version of brewer's yeast that can aid in the production of significant amounts of lactic acid in the intestine. The additional acid can work quickly and when taken with probiotic supplements can do wonders for your gut. You can chew one of these lactic acid yeast wafers each meal. In most cases, this product is only needed for 5-7 days and you can continue taking probiotic supplements.

When there are carbohydrates in our stomach that can't be digested, these bacteria help to ferment them. Results from this process of fermentation help keep the gut acidic and keep harmful microorganism to grow as good bacteria. Also, it helps to eat twice daily with your meals.

When traditional fermented foods aren't available, you can take probiotic supplements instead to get the benefits of probiotic bacteria. This is also a convenient way to take probiotics for people on travel or for those who simply can't take eating fermented foods.

Consider Intermittent Fasting

Consider fasting on 16-24 hours timeframes or twice a week as it gives the gastrointestinal tract a needed rest from the burden of food processing and digestion. If you opt for the liquid diet route, then you have got to stick to bone broth, meat and fish stock, vegetables, and fresh vegetable juices. These liquids are nutrient-packed and gentle to leaky gut.

Practice Meditation

Meditation is an excellent combatant for stress and in our current lifestyle, we are constantly bombarded with pressure. While we are very much aware that chronic stress is one of the major causes of the leaky gut due to its crippling effect on the digestive system, it would be tough for your body to fight against bad bacteria and yeast overgrowth. This leads to gut permeability along with inflammation flares associated with leaky gut.

Meditation is now considered a complementary mind-body medicine that produces a deep state of relaxation and tranquil state of mind. A 10-minute meditation a day that involves deep breathing can do much to release stress and doing this slows down the part of your nervous system that inhibits digestion. It likewise activates the hormones that aids in digestion.

Do Some Exercise

Doing exercises stimulates the nerves to help maintain mobility of the gut. A sedentary lifestyle can contribute to a neurological slow down of the gut function.

Take High-Quality Probiotics

Probiotics aids in indigestion and regulates your immune responses. You need at least 80 billion CFU (colony forming unit). CFU is the measurement used in probiotics for good and bad bacteria, including yeast.

Doing a Leaky Test

Leaky gut symptoms can be like symptoms of other major illnesses. To be sure, visit your doctor and have it diagnosed adequately through a leak test. Also, have your doctor test you for other hidden allergies. This will help you get rid of potential sources of food-based inflammation and persistent gut damage.

Treat Intestinal Pathogens

A variety of parasites can cause infection to the intestinal tract. Parasites are acquired when you have consumed contaminated food or water. People with imbalanced gut flora, leaky gut syndrome or weakened immune response system are more susceptible to parasites. There are natural ways of cleansing these parasites.

- Take three times a day of 250 milligrams of black walnuts. This had been mentioned in history to be useful in the treatment of parasites.

- Wormwood is known for its anti-parasitic properties. Consuming 200 ml. of wormwood, three times in a day can help you get rid of these parasites. However, consider utmost caution in its dosage as large dose can be toxic.

- Oregano oil has both antibacterial and anti-parasitic effects. Take 500 milligrams of the oil 4x daily.

- Grapefruit seed extract has anti-parasitic effects and you should take it as directed based on the supplier's instruction provided with the item.

Consider Including Whole Foods in your Diet

Whole foods are foods in their most natural state or they are closest to the way nature delivers them. It means, they are minimally processed and without any additives. Most foods that are organic are also probiotics and therefore helpful in creating a balance in your gut flora. Fresh fruits and vegetables are some of best whole foods recommended for one suffering from a leaky gut.

The Gut-Counteractive Diet Plan

	Breakfast	Lunch	Dinner	Snacks
Monday	Bacon, Chicken and Pecan Salad	The Ultimate Healthy Gut Noodles	Stir-fried Gingered Salmon	Mixed Fruits Yogurt (lactose-free)

Tuesday	Smoked Salmon Breakfast Delight Quick and Easy Back Rice Mix	Bone Broth Roasted Potatoes	Cucumber and Crab Salad	Turkey Tortilla Sandwich
Wednesday	Vegetable Juice Coconut yogurt with fruits Turkey Sausage (Gluten/Soy-Free)	Herb-Crusted Salmon Boiled Rice	Mixed Vegetables Lamb chops Sauerkraut	Green Smoothie

Thursday	Oat Porridge with Fruit Delight Lemon water/ juice	Bacon & Brie Omelet Wedges with Summer Salad	Steamed Artichoke with sea salt and lemon juice	Apple or any fruit of your choice
Friday	Meaty Zucchini with Onions and Mushrooms	Coconut Chicken with Spinach	Spicy Shrimp-Avocado Turret	Cucumber with salt Herbal tea
Saturday	Stir-Fried Gingered Salmon	Italian - Style Pan Fried Broccoli	Vegetable Stew	Herbal Tea Mixed Fruits

| Sunday | Superfood for Gut Burger | Lemony Omelet with Smoked | Salmon and Spinach with Tartare Cream | Zucchini Noodles |

Chapter 5: Bounce Back to Life with Gut-Healthy Recipes

The Bone Broth and Other Soup Recipes

Recipe #1 - Bone Broth

Servings: 2-4

Ingredients

- 4 Pounds beef bones
- 2 tbsp. Apple cider vinegar
- 12 cups Water
- 1 1/2 cups carrots (chopped)
- 1 1/2 cups leeks (chopped)
- 3-5 sprigs Fresh rosemary
- 1 tsp. Black peppercorns

- 3 Bay leaves

- 6 cloves of garlic

- 1 medium-sized Onion (Roughly diced)

Directions

1. Preheat the oven to 450 degrees Fahrenheit and prepare a baking sheet lined with aluminum foil. Arrange the bones on the baking sheet and roast for about 40 minutes, flipping once to ensure even cooking on both sides.

2. When bones are cooked, place them in a large stockpot with water. Add in vinegar and allow to sit at room temperature for approximately 30 minutes.

3. Roughy chops vegetables before adding to the stockpot. Bring it to boil and when it does reach the boiling point, lower down the heat and let it simmer. For 2-3 hours, discard the foamy formation on top of the soup.

4. You may simmer it for 48 hours for beef bone broth, 24 hours for chicken bone broth, and 8 hours for fish bone broth.

5. Allow to cool slightly and strain. Pour the broth into an airtight container. Refrigerate for about4-6 hours or overnight. This will allow the fat to rise to allow the fat settle to the top and solidify.

6. Scrape the fat off the top with a spoon. This will leave you with a gelatinous bone broth when cold.

7. Store in an airtight mason jar or freeze until ready to use. When ready to use, slowly warm the broth over a low heat to bring it back to a liquid consistency.

NUTRITIONAL FACTS	
Serving Size	1 cup
Calories	160 cal
Fats	12 g
Carbohydrates	2 g
Protein	6 g

Recipe #2 - Chicken Zoodle Bone Broth Soup

Servings: 2-4

Ingredients

For the bone broth:

- Whole organic chicken
- 6 cloves garlic
- 1 onion
- 1 inch of ginger root

For the soup:

- 4-6 cups Organic chicken broth
- 2 tbsp. Coconut oil
- 1-2 cups chopped onions
- 1-2 cups chopped carrots
- 3-4 small to medium zucchinis

- 2 cups shredded organic chicken

- 2 to 3 garlic cloves, crushed or minced

- Himalayan sea salt to taste

Directions

Bone Broth:

1. Clean the chicken and put it in the pot. Then fill it with water up to three-quarters full before adding herbs and vegetables.

2. Cook over medium-high heat it boils, then reduce heat and allow to simmer, covered for about 8-48 hours depending on your desire.

3. Allow cooling before passing the stock through a strainer and transferring to Mason jars for storage. Keep it in the fridge.

Soup:

1. In a pan, sauté the onions and carrots using coconut oil.

2. When onions become translucent, add bone broth and bring to a boil.

3. Make noodles from zucchini and slice it into strips of desired sizes. You can also use a julienne slicer for this.

4. Add zucchini when carrots become tender and leave to simmer.

5. Add in garlic and chopped chicken. Cook until it boils and then turns the heat off. Cover and allow to sit for 5-10 minutes.

NUTRITIONAL FACTS	
Serving Size	1 cup
Calories	53 cal
Fats	0.3 g
Carbohydrates	0.7 g
Protein	6 g

Recipe #3 - Herb Roasted Bone Marrow

Servings: 1-2

Ingredients

- Fresh Rosemary

- Fresh thyme

- Marrow bones of grass-fed or pasture-raised beef

- Unrefined salt and black pepper to taste

Directions

1. Thaw the bones when frozen.

2. Prepare the other even by preheating to 400/degrees Fahrenheit. Arrange bones in the baking dish.

3. Finely chop fresh thyme and rosemary and sprinkle them as over bones.

4. Roast bones for about 15 minutes until there are no more visible pink residues on the inside of the bones, but make sure you don't cook long enough to have marrows cookout to leave the bone casing.

5. Season with salt and pepper and serve hot.

NUTRITIONAL FACTS	
Serving Size	1 oz.
Calories	37 cal
Fats	2.5 g
Carbohydrates	0.2 g
Protein	3.1 g

Recipe #4 - Homemade Beef Broth

Servings: 1-2

Ingredients

- 2.5 lbs. of marrow bones
- 2.5 lbs. of soft bones
- Juice extracted from half lemon fruit or a few drops of apple cider vinegar.
- 2 tbsp. Parsley
- 2 tbsp. Sea salt
- 2 tbsp. Black pepper
- Vegetables (optional)

Directions

1. Add all bones into a stock pot or slow cooker.
2. Add a few shots of apple cider vinegar or lemon juice.

3. Fill the pot with filtered water but not enough to have it spilled out when boiling. Set to slow cooking over low heat for 24/hours.

4. After 24 hours, you may add some vegetables for flavor. You may choose carrots, sweet onions, celery stalks along with salt and pepper to taste. Make sure you remove veggies before they are overcooked.

5. Then set for another 12 hours or depends on your preference but the longer you cook, the more nutrients are released into the broth.

6. After 30 hours, check to see if the marrow had fallen out of the bones. After 30 hours of slow cooking, turn off heat and let it cool off.

7. When cool, drain broth using a mesh colander.

8. Store it in the fridge for supply and serve hot when needed.4 cups mussels, cut into chunks.

NUTRITIONAL FACTS	
Serving Size	2 cups
Calories	250 g
Fats	5 g
Carbohydrates	2 g
Protein	3 g

Recipe #5 - Thai Carrot Soup

Serving: 1-2

Ingredients

- 1 large onion, diced

- About 1-inch slice of fresh ginger, peeled and grated (about 1 tsp.).

- 1 1/2 tsp. curry powder

- 2 tbsps. of olive oil, coconut oil, or ghee

- 3 to 4 cups broth or water

- 1/4 cup coconut milk (or other milk)

- 2 pounds carrots, peeled and chopped into coins

- 1/2 tsp. salt

- 1 to 2 tsp. of fresh lemon juice (optional)

Directions

1. Place a stock pot over medium heat to keep it warm. When warm, add the oil, then onions and book for 5-19 minutes until they appear translucent.

2. Add spices and salt to coat onions evenly.

3. Add stock or water along with carrots

4. Bring soup to book and allow to simmer for about 15 minutes until carrots become tender.

5. Serve while hot.

NUTRITIONAL FACTS	
Serving Size	1 cup
Calories	170 cal
Fats	12 g
Carbohydrates	16 g
Protein	1 g

Recipe #6 - Mussels Soup

Servings 6

Ingredients

- 4 cups mussels, cut into chunks
- 6 cups bone broth
- 2 jalapenos, seeded and sliced
- 1 tbsp. cilantro
- 1 tbsp. parsley
- 4 tbsp. coconut oil

*Add your favorite vegetables, herbs, and spices

Directions

1. Pour broth into a large pot and allow it to simmer over low heat. Then add jalapenos, parsley, and cilantro into the pot.

2. Also, add mussels and coconut oil. Let it simmer until mussels shells are opened.

3. Ladle soup into bowls and serve.

NUTRITIONAL FACTS	
Serving Size	1 cup
Calories	80 cal
Fats	2.2 g
Carbohydrates	2.5 g
Protein	16 g

Recipe #7 - Creamy Potato and Chicken Soup

Serving: 1-2

Ingredients

- 1 onion, chopped
- 3 stalks celery, chopped
- 12 oz. package nitrate free bacon, diced
- 4 cloves garlic, minced
- 2 bay leaves
- 6 cups white sweet potatoes, peeled and cubed
- 8 cups chicken bone broth
- 5-7 cups cooked chicken, shredded
- 6 cups parsnips, peeled and cubed (or rutabaga or combination of both)
- 1 leek (see note on preparation below)
- juice of one large lemon (maybe more)

- 2 carrots, chopped

- salt and pepper to taste

- sliced green onions, optional

Directions

1. Start by preparing the leek. Cut it in half lengthwise and slice thinly. Place slices of leeks in a bowl of cold water. After à few seconds, take it out of the water and drain.

2. Preheat a large pot or Dutch oven to medium and add the bacon and stir a little until crispy. Remove the bacon from the pot and drain on paper towels and set aside.

3. Add onions, celery, leeks, and carrots to bacon in a pot with grease. Cook and stir until soft. Add garlic and stir more for 30 seconds.

4. Add white potatoes, bay leaves, bone broth, and parsnips. Cook until root veggies are cooked and tender.

5. Remove the bay leaf. Ladle about a third or half of the soup into a high-powered blender. Make sure you include the broth and root veggies. Puree until soft. You may likewise use an immersion blender if available so can do the blending right there in the pot.

6. Once pureed, put the soup back into the pot and stir. Note that the soup thickens and become creamy.

7. Next, add salt and pepper to taste along with lemon juice. Stir well and suit to taste.

8. Add shredded chicken and stir again.

9. Serve with bacon and green onions for garnishing.

NUTRITIONAL FACTS	
Serving Size	1 cup
Calories	155 cal
Fats	4 g
Carbohydrates	41 g
Protein	8 g

Recipe #8 - Chicken Zoodle Faux Pho

Serving: 1

Ingredients

- 2 Garlic cloves, crushed
- ⅓ cup Green onion, chopped fine
- 1 tbsp. Oil
- 2 cups Mushrooms (preferably Shiitake), sliced
- 4 cups Chicken bone broth
- ½ cup Coconut milk
- 2 tsp. Ginger, grated
- 2 tbsp. Freshly squeezed lime juice
- 1 tbsp. Red Boat fish sauce
- 1-2 Carrots, peeled and shredded ¼ c chopped cilantro
- 1 lb. Skinless, boneless chicken, cubed

- 2 cups Zucchini noodles

Directions

1. In a large pot, heat oil over medium heat.

2. Saute garlic, ginger, mushrooms, onions, and shredded carrot for about 3 minutes.

3. Then add broth, fish sauce, and coconut milk.

4. Bring to boil and then reduce heat while allowing it to simmer.

5. Add the chicken and let it simmer for another 7-10 minutes.

Recipe #9 - Crock Pot Pho

Serving: 2

Ingredients

For the Pho Stock:

- Half Onion
- 4 pounds beef bones
- 2 1/2 tablespoons fish sauce or to taste
- 4-inch section of ginger, sliced
- 16 ounces fresh or dried rice noodles
- 9 cups water
- 1 teaspoon sugar
- 1 package Vietnamese Pho Spices or prepare these spices: 2 cinnamon sticks, 1 tsp. of fennel, 2 tsp. Of whole coriander, 3 whole cloves, 3 whole star anise, and 1 cardamom pod

For the Pho Bowls:

- 11 ounces Vietnamese beef balls, cut into half
- 1/2 pound flank, London broil, sirloin or eye of round steak, sliced as thinly as possible.
- For the table
- 2 big handfuls of bean sprouts
- 2-3 chili peppers, sliced
- fresh herbs: cilantro, Thai basil, mint
- Sriracha hot chili sauce
- 1-2 limes, cut into wedges
- Hoisin sauce

Directions

1. Boil water in a large stockpot over high heat. When it starts to boil, add the beef bones and continue with the boiling for about 10 minutes.

2. Simultaneously, preheat frying pan over medium-low heat. Add in Vietnamese Pho Spices and toast for about 2-3 minutes or until aroma comes out. Pace the spices to a crockpot or slow cooker. Return the frying pan over medium-high heat and add a tablespoon of oil. Once the oil is hot, add slices of ginger and half of the onion. Flip to brown both sides. Add the onion and ginger to the crockpot.

3. Drain and discard water from the pre-boiled bones and rinse them to clean. Add bones to the crockpot or slow cooker and fi it with fresh water - about 1 ½ inches just below the surface. Then also, add the sugar and fish. With lid cover, set to slow cook for about 8 hours. Taste and season.

4. When ready, prepare the rest of the ingredients for the Pho bowls. Boil a pot of water and add the beef balls as soon as it reaches the boiling point and cooks for around 2 minutes. Remove balls while the water keeps on boiling. Cook the noodles as per package

instruction. When using fresh noodles, add a couple of minutes to boiling and then drain.

5. Prepare 4 large empty bowls on the counter and fill it with noodles, beef base, and thin steak slices evenly divided among the bowls. Ladle Pho stock into each bowl and make sure that the stock is hot enough to cook the thin steak slices before serving. Garnish with lime wedges, chili peppers, and fresh herbs. Also, served with Hoisin sauce and Sriracha chili sauce.

NUTRITIONAL FACTS	
Serving Size	1 cup
Calories	340 cal
Fats	15 g
Carbohydrates	3 g
Protein	20 g

Recipe #10 - Creamy Broccoli Soup

Serving: 2

Ingredients

- 2 cloves garlic

- 1 potato, peeled and roughly chopped into cubes about 1.5cm / ½" cubes

- 1 cup milk (low fat, cow or soy)

- 2 cups vegetable stock/broth

- 1 white or brown onion, roughly diced

- 1 large head of broccoli

- ½ cup water

- Salt and pepper

Directions

1. Break broccoli florets into pieces. Discard the main stem and cut the other stems into pieces the size of a thumb.

2. Put ingredients except milk, pepper, and salt in a pot and cover to boil. Once boiling, reduce heat to medium and allow to simmer for 8-10 minutes.

3. Remove the lid cover, add in milk, then bring back to boil. Remove from heat and whizz it using a manual bender.

4. Cooking it longer under medium will thicken the sauce. Season to taste.

NUTRITIONAL FACTS	
Serving Size	1 cup
Calories	300 cal
Fats	22 g
Carbohydrates	18 g
Protein	4 g

Detoxifying Smoothies, Juices, and Other Drinks

Recipe #11- Natural Ginger Ale

This old-fashioned ginger ale is naturally fermented and filled with beneficial probiotics and enzymes to help you maintain your gut health or repair a leaky gut.

Servings: 1

Ingredients

- 1 piece of ginger (about 1-2 inches)
- ½ cup Organic sugar or add molasses if you use regular sugar
- ½ tsp. Sea salt or Himalayan salt
- ½ cup of Fresh lemon extract or lime juice
- ½ cup of Filtered water (Chlorine-free)
- ½ cup of homemade ginger bug or ¼ cup of whey

NUTRITIONAL FACTS	
Serving Size	1 bottle
Calories	170 cal
Fats	0 g
Carbohydrates	42 g
Protein	0 g

Recipe #12- Coconut Water Kefir

Servings: 1

Ingredients

- 4 cups of coconut water

- ¼ cup of kefir starter or water kefir grains

Directions

1. In a mason jar, mix all ingredients and set on a counter. Leave it there for 1-2 days. After 7 days, check on the coconut water kefir. Taste and if it turns sour then it's ready. If still sweet, leave it for another day.

2. Store it in the refrigerator and serve cold. Add a squeeze of lemon juice for added flavor.

NUTRITIONAL FACTS	
Serving Size	100 ml
Calories	28 cal
Fats	0 g
Carbohydrates	0.5 g
Protein	0.2 g

Recipe #13 - Orange Juice Detox

Servings: 1

Ingredients

- Extract from a freshly squeezed orange juice
- Filtered water
- 1/2 tsp Culture Starter or 2 tbsp whey
- Sea Salt

Directions

1. Prepare about 2 ½ cups of freshly squeezed orange juice
2. Add ½ teaspoon of culture starter or about 2 tablespoons of whey. Add a pinch of salt.
3. Fill the jar with a cup of water (at room Temperature and filtered). Leave about an inch space.

4. Cover it and give a quick shake. Leave it for about 48 hours at room temperature.

5. Cool it in the fridge and enjoy!

NUTRITIONAL FACTS	
Serving Size	1 cup
Calories	59 cal
Fats	0 g
Carbohydrates	14 g
Protein	1 g

Recipe #14 - Gut-Soothing Ginger & Slippery Elm Tea

Servings: 1

Ingredients

- 1 tsp. Slippery elm powder
- 1 tsp. Fresh ginger root
- 2 cups Purified water

Directions

1. Grate your fresh ginger and pace in your teapot.
2. Add 2 cups of water and bring to boil.
3. Pass through a strainer to separate residues.
4. Add slippery elm powder and stir.

NUTRITIONAL FACTS	
Serving Size	1 tsp.
Calories	5 cal
Fats	0 g
Carbohydrates	1.2 g
Protein	0 g

Recipe #15 - Gut-Healing Smoothie

Servings: 1

Ingredients

- 1-2 cups Full-fat coconut milk or almond milk
- 2 Frozen bananas, cut into chunks
- 1 tbsp, Freshly grated ginger
- 1/2 tbsp. Bee pollen
- 1/2 tbsp. Chia or flax seeds
- 2 tbsp. collagen protein or whey protein
- 2 cups Spinach
- 2 cups kale
- 1/2 Avocado
- 1 tbsp. Hemp hearts
- 1 tbsp. Raw honey or manuka honey

Directions

Place ingredients in a blender and bend high on high until smooth (about 2-3 minutes).

Serve with ice.

NUTRITIONAL FACTS	
Serving Size	2 cups
Calories	375 cal
Fats	40 g
Carbohydrates	26 g
Protein	13 g

Recipe #16 - Anti-Inflammatory Turmeric Milk

Servings: 1

Ingredients

- ½-3/4 tsp. ginger
- ½ cup coconut cream with an added ½ cup of filtered water or 1 cup of coconut milk
- 1 to 2 tsp. honey to taste
- ½-3/4 tsp. turmeric
- Dash of freshly ground pepper
- Other possible additions:
- ¼ tsp. cinnamon
- ½ tsp. cardamom

Directions

1. In a saucepan, heat over low-medium heat the coconut cream and water/coconut milk, turmeric,

ginger, and ground pepper until it simmer. Remove from heat and allow mixture to settle for 10-20 minutes for flavor to be enhanced.

2. Reheat until warm enough but not hot and add honey to taste. Enjoy!

NUTRITIONAL FACTS	
Serving Size	12 oz.
Calories	130 cal
Fats	1 g
Carbohydrates	30.1 g
Protein	3.7 g

Recipe #17 - Cilantro - Cucumber Juice

Servings: 1

Ingredients

- 1-inch of ginger root
- 1 jicama
- 1 cucumber
- 1 lime
- A handful of cilantro
- 2 ounces of Aloe vera (optional)

NUTRITIONAL FACTS	
Serving Size	1 cucumber
Calories	28 cal
Fats	0.3 g
Carbohydrates	7.7 g
Protein	1.4 g

Recipe #18 - Cucumber Mint Drink

Servings: 1

Ingredients

- 1 cucumber

- ½ head of fennel

- 2 handfuls of mint leaves

- ½ lemon

NUTRITIONAL FACTS	
Serving Size	2.24 oz.
Calories	35 cal
Fats	0 g
Carbohydrates	8 g
Protein	0 g

Recipe #19 - Revitalizing Papaya Smoothie

Servings: 1

Ingredients

- ½ a small papaya

- 1 banana

- 1 lemon wedge

NUTRITIONAL FACTS	
Serving Size	1 ¼ cup
Calories	176 cal
Fats	1 g
Carbohydrates	42 g
Protein	3 g

Recipe #20 - Go Green Gut Recipe

Servings: 1

Ingredients

- 1 cucumber

- 1-inch slice ginger

- 1 head fennel

- 1-2 handfuls mint leaves

- ½-1 lemon (optional)

How to Make Fruit/Vegetable Juice/Smoothie

- Clean each fruit and vegetables to use. Remove cores and skin if needed before cutting them into small pieces. Dicing fruits into inch cubes will make it easier to blend and maximize juice extraction. For hard fruits like apples, add a half cup of water for every four apples. You may add more water later when using traditional blender or smoothie blender when needed according to consistency desired.

- Place hard ingredients first and bend on puree setting for a few hours. Then add other ingredients and continue blending until you reach desired consistency. Place in the fridge to cool before serving.

NUTRITIONAL FACTS	
Serving Size	1 cup
Calories	40 cal
Fats	0 g
Carbohydrates	8 g
Protein	2 g

Anti-Leak Food Recipes for the Gut

Recipe #21- Superfood for Gut Burger

Servings:

Ingredients

- 1¼ lbs. Grass-fed ground beef
- ¼ cup Organic mustard
- ½ cup Drained organic sauerkraut
- ½ head Organic lettuce
- ½ cup Watercress
- ½ a White organic onion, sliced
- Himalayan sea salt to taste

Direction

1. Heat grill to medium-high. Form the beef into four ¾-inch-thick patties. Season with salt.

2. Cook the patties until desired readiness.

3. Use the lettuce leaves as the "sandwich buns" and add the burgers, onion, watercress, mustard, and sauerkraut.

Benefits: You'll obtain good anti-inflammatory fats like CLA and omegas from the grass-fed burger, probiotics, and phytonutrients from the vegetables, and good bacteria from the sauerkraut, all in one meal!

NUTRITIONAL FACTS	
Serving Size	1 burger
Calories	40 cal
Fats	3 g
Carbohydrates	5 g
Protein	2 g

Recipe #22 - Herb-Crusted Salmon

Servings:

Ingredients

For the salmon:

- 2 x 6oz. Salmon fillets
- 1 tbsp. Coconut flour
- 2 tbsp. Fresh or dried parsley
- 1 tbsp. Dijon mustard
- 1 tbsp. Olive oil
- Salt and pepper

For the salad:

- 2 cups Arugula
- ¼ Red onion, thinly sliced

- 1 tbsp. White wine vinegar

- Juice of 1 Lemon

- 1 tbsp. Olive oil

- Salt and pepper

Directions

1. Preheat the oven to 450°F.

2. Meanwhile, put the fish on a baking sheet lined with aluminum foil or parchment paper.

3. Top the fish with mustard and olive oil then rub it into the fillets.

4. Mix the flour, parsley, salt and pepper in a small bowl.

5. Using a spoon, sprinkle the mixture to the fillets. Gently pat them to the fillets.

6. Cook for about 10-15 minutes or according to your desired doneness.

7. While cooking the fillets, mix all the salad ingredients in a large salad bowl.

8. Once the fillets are done, top them with the salad and serve.

NUTRITIONAL FACTS	
Serving Size	1 fillet
Calories	455 cal
Fats	22.7 g
Carbohydrates	12 g
Protein	33 g

Recipe #23 - Gut-Friendly Breakfast Scramble

Servings: 4

Ingredients

- 8 oz. Ground pork or lamb
- 10 Cherry tomatoes halved
- 2 cup Hearty greens (like collards, chard or black kale)
- 1 cup Carrots or sweet potato, shredded
- 4 Eggs whisked
- Sea salt and pepper
- Avocado, scallions or chives—for garnish

Directions

1. In a nonstick skillet, brown the pork or lamb over medium heat. Add the shredded carrots (or sweet

potato) plus the greens. Continue to cook for about 3 minutes or until the greens have wilted. Place the tomatoes and stir for about half a minute.

2. Lower the heat to medium-low, add the whisked eggs and stir. Season with salt and pepper. Top with preferred garnish and serve.

NUTRITIONAL FACTS	
Serving Size	1 cup
Calories	208 cal
Fats	57 g
Carbohydrates	30 g
Protein	51 g

Recipe #24 - Coconut Chicken Curry

Servings: 1

Ingredients

- 1 Chicken breast, cooked and cut into bite-sized pieces
- 1 x 13.5 oz. can full-fat coconut milk
- 1 tbsp. olive oil
- 1 Sweet potato, peeled and chopped into half cubes
- 2 Cloves garlic, chopped
- ½ cup Green onions, chopped
- ½ tbsp. Turmeric
- 1 tbsp. Coriander
- ½ tbsp. Cumin
- ½ tsp. Onion powder
- Onion, diced

- Celery stalks, chopped

- 1 cup Water

- 1 tsp. Salt

- 1 Avocado, sliced—for garnish

Directions

1. Place a large skillet over medium heat and pour oil.

2. Add the chopped garlic and brown them slightly.

3. Add the onions, pour more oil (if you want to), and cook until the onions are translucent.

4. Next, add the onion powder, cumin, turmeric, and coriander. Mix the herbs and add the potatoes, celery, and green onions.

5. Pour a cup of water and a teaspoon of salt. Boil until the potatoes are tender.

6. Add the chicken and coconut milk. Let it simmer for several minutes.

7. Top with avocado slices before serving.

NUTRITIONAL FACTS	
Serving Size	1 cup
Calories	421 cal
Fats	26.6 g
Carbohydrates	11.2 g
Protein	36.1 g

Recipe #25 - Bacon-Packed Potatoes

Servings: 1

Ingredients

- 2 cups Fresh spinach
- 2 Medium sweet potatoes, cooked, warmed and halved
- 1 Large sweet onion, sliced
- 4 Slices bacon
- 1 Avocado, cubed
- 1 Scallion, chopped
- 3 Cloves garlic, sliced
- 1 tbsp. Coconut oil

Directions

1. Put a large skillet over medium heat and crisp the bacon slices. Once cooked, transfer to a plate and set aside. Don't remove the grease from the pan.

2. Put a tablespoon of coconut oil in the pan and add the garlic and onions. Cook over medium heat, stirring frequently until the onions have caramelized. Remove the garlic-onion mixture from the pan and set aside.

3. Place the spinach in the skillet and cook until leaves have wilted.

4. Arrange the sliced potatoes on a serving plate. Garnish them with the caramelized onion-garlic mixture, half of the spinach, two bacon slices, and half of the avocado. Serve while still warm.

NUTRITIONAL FACTS	
Serving Size	1 cup
Calories	340 cal
Fats	14.6 g
Carbohydrates	38.2 g
Protein	14.6 g

Recipe#26 - Meaty Zucchini with Onions and Mushrooms

Servings: 1

Ingredients

- 1 small Zucchini, thinly sliced
- 1 lb. Ground bison
- 1 Small white onion, thinly sliced
- 3 tbsp. Coconut flour
- 1 tbsp. Dried basil
- 1 tbsp. Onion powder
- 1 tbsp. Garlic powder1 tsp sea salt
- 2 tbsp. Kalamata olive tapenade—optional
- 10 Button mushrooms, sliced thinly—optional

Directions

1. Preheat oven to 400°F.

2. In a medium mixing bowl, put together the ground bison, white onion, onion powder, dried basil, garlic powder, and salt. Set aside.

3. In the bottom of a glass baking dish or large cast iron skillet, press the meat mixture as thinly as possible.

4. Top the meat mixture with the olive spread in one, thin layer. Next, evenly distribute the zucchini, onion, and mushroom slices.

5. Bake for about 25 minutes or until veggies are tender and the meat is cooked through.

NUTRITIONAL FACTS	
Serving Size	1 slice
Calories	411 cal
Fats	17 g
Carbohydrates	41 g
Protein	23 g

Recipe #27 - Turkey Tortilla Sandwich

Servings: 2

Ingredients

- 8 slices turkey lunch meat, sliced thinly

- 2 grain-free tortillas (plus 2 more if desired)

- 4 romaine lettuce leaves

- ½ cup alfalfa sprouts ½ cup shredded carrots

- 1 avocado, pitted and sliced

- 2 tbsp. organic apple cider vinegar mustard

Directions

1. In a dry pan, warm the tortillas until they're bendy.

2. Distribute half of the avocado slices over the tortillas and spread the mustard over them.

3. On top of the avocado-mustard mixture, place four turkey slices per tortilla.

4. Place the lettuce leaves on top of the turkey slices, to be followed by the carrots and sprouts.

5. Fold the tortillas in half or feel free to use another one per tortilla to cover.

NUTRITIONAL FACTS	
Serving Size	1 sandwich
Calories	285.7 cal
Fats	12.6 g
Carbohydrates	26.6 g
Protein	16.5 g

Recipe #28- Cucumber and Crab Salad

Servings: 2

Ingredients

- 5 oz. lump crab meat, cooked and chilled
- 1 cucumber, thinly sliced
- 2 celery stalks, thinly sliced
- ¼ cup red onion, thinly sliced
- 2 tbsp. coconut nectar
- 2 tbsp. coconut aminos
- 2 tbsp. lemon juice
- 1 tbsp. toasted sesame oil
- 12 oz. kelp noodles—optional

Directions

1. Add all the ingredients together in a large salad bowl. Toss everything together to combine.

2. Add the kelp noodles and chill before serving.

NUTRITIONAL FACTS	
Serving Size	1 cup
Calories	201 cal
Fats	6 g
Carbohydrates	11 g
Protein	26 g

Recipe #29 - Simple Broccoli Salad

Servings: 2

Ingredients

- 3 cups broccoli florets
- 2 cups broccoli stems, grated
- 1 cup paleo mayonnaise
- ½ cup golden raisins
- ½ cup green onions, chopped
- ½ cup sunflower seeds
- 2 tbsp. red wine vinegar

Directions

1. Mix the green onions, golden raisins, sunflower seeds, broccoli florets, and grated stems and in a large salad bowl.

2. Add the vinegar and stir.

3. Add the mayonnaise and mix until well combined. Chill before serving.

NUTRITIONAL FACTS	
Serving Size	1 cup
Calories	25 g
Fats	0 g
Carbohydrates	4 g
Protein	2 g

Recipe #30 - Israeli Salad with Grilled Chicken

Servings: 2

Ingredients

- 1 English cucumber, chopped
- 2 Extra large tomatoes, chopped
- 1 Red bell pepper, chopped
- 1 Yellow bell pepper, chopped
- ½ Medium red onion, chopped
- ½ cup Herbs*, chopped
- 4 tbsp. Olive oil
- Juice of ½ lemon (or more to taste)
- Zest of one lemon
- Salt and pepper
- Grilled chicken, for serving

*Note: You can choose from Italian parsley, cilantro, mint or a mixture of these.

Directions

Place all the ingredients together in a large salad bowl. Toss until fully combined.

Serve with grilled chicken.

NUTRITIONAL FACTS	
Serving Size	1 gram
Calories	204 cal
Fats	15 g
Carbohydrates	3 g
Protein	13 g

Recipe #31 - Lemony Omelet with Smoked Trout

Servings: 2

Ingredients

- 5 Free range eggs
- 200g Smoked trout fillet
- 2 tsp Lemon juice
- 1 tsp Lemon zest
- 1 tbs. Ghee or coconut oil
- Salt and pepper
- 2 Lemon wedges, for serving

Direction

1. Whisk the eggs, lemon juice and zest in a bowl.
2. Heat a skillet over medium-high flame and heat the ghee or coconut oil.

3. Add the eggs and cook until they're soft.

4. Season with salt and pepper. Serve with smoked trout and lemon wedges on the side.

NUTRITIONAL FACTS	
Serving Size	100 grams
Calories	206 cal
Fats	8 g
Carbohydrates	0.4 g
Protein	31.3 g

Recipe #32 - Zucchini Noodles

Servings: 2

Ingredients

- 2 Large zucchini washed and patted dry
- 1 tbs. Coconut oil or ghee
- Sea salt and pepper

Directions

1. Cut the zucchini into thin strips with a mandolin slicer to make "noodles."

2. Put the noodles in a sieve and generously sprinkle with sea salt. Set it aside for about 20 minutes or until the moisture has been removed from the noodles.

3. After the allotted time, pat the noodles dry with paper towel.

4. Place pan on a medium heat and melt the ghee. Once hot, add the noodles and toss for about a minute or two until cooked through.

5. Serve with your favorite pasta sauce.

NUTRITIONAL FACTS	
Serving Size	4 oz.
Calories	90 cal
Fats	8 g
Carbohydrates	4 g
Protein	1 g

Recipe #33 - Healthy Gut Zesty Salad with Fish Cakes

Servings: 2

Ingredients

For the fish cakes:

- 750g Whitefish, diced
- 2 eggs
- 4 Spring onions (green part only), sliced
- 1 Long red chili, minced
- 1 ½ cups Macadamia nuts
- 1 Garlic clove, minced
- 1 tbs. Apple cider vinegar
- 1 tbs. Coconut oil
- 1 tbs. Lime juice

For the salad:

- 4 Iceberg lettuce leaves
- ½ Large cucumber, sliced
- A handful of Cherry tomatoes
- A handful of Vietnamese mint
- 2 tbsp. Olive oil
- 2 tbsp. Lime juice
- 1 Lime, halved

Directions

1. Put the fish, 1 egg, spring onions, ginger, chili, garlic, and lime juice in a food processor. Process until you get a smooth texture.

2. In a bowl, whisk the other egg. On a plate, put the macadamia nuts.

3. Remove the fish mixture from the processor and form them into patties.

4. Dip one patty in the whisked egg, roll it in the nuts and then place it on a plate. Do this step to all the patties.

5. Place pan over medium heat and melt the ghee. Once hot, fry the fishcakes until cooked through.

6. For the salad, add all the ingredients—except for the halved lime—in a large salad bowl and toss. Season to taste.

7. Serve the salad with the fishcakes on top and the lime halves on the side.

NUTRITIONAL FACTS	
Serving Size	1 cake
Calories	175 ca
Fats	6.5 g
Carbohydrates	26.5 g
Protein	5g

Recipe #34 - Bacon, Chicken and Pecan Salad

Servings: 2

Ingredients

For the salad:

- 1 ½ cups Free-range chicken, cooked and diced
- 2 cups Mixed salad leaves, washed and drained
- 4 Rashers free-range, nitrate and sugar-free bacon
- 20 Raw and activated pecans
- 1 Red capsicum, diced

For the dressing:

- 2 tbsp. Lemon juice
- 2 tbsp. Olive oil
- Salt and pepper

Directions

1. Put a skillet over medium heat and cook the bacon. Once cool, chop them into bits.

2. Toss the chicken, salad leaves, bacon bits, pecans, and capsicum in a large salad bowl.

3. In a small bowl, mix the lemon juice and olive oil. Season with salt and pepper.

4. Drizzle the salad with dressing and toss again. Serve.

NUTRITIONAL FACTS	
Serving Size	1 minimal share
Calories	667.9 ca
Fats	42.3 g
Carbohydrates	27.3 g
Protein	46.1

Recipe #35 - Spanish Sausage and Baked Eggs

Servings:

Ingredients

- 2 Spanish-style sausages, gluten-free and nitrate-free
- 6 Free-range eggs
- 1 cup Broccoli florets
- 1 red Capsicum, diced
- 1 tsp. Ground coriander
- 1 tsp. Cumin
- 1 tsp. Paprika
- 1 tsp. Ghee or tallow

Directions

1. Preheat oven to 350°F.

2. Place an oven-safe, nonstick pan over medium heat. Heat oil and melt the ghee. Remove the skin of sausages and cook.

3. When the sausages are nearly cooked through, add the capsicum and cook for 2 minutes. Add the broccoli and continue to cook for another 2 minutes.

4. Stir in the cumin, coriander, and paprika.

5. Add the eggs. Make sure that they poured evenly, so they cover the base of the pan. Continue to cook for another 2 minutes before moving it to the oven.

6. Cook in the oven for about 10 minutes. You will know that it's done once the whites are already firm. (If you want a hard yolk, leave the pan for a few more minutes.) Serve with the salad on the side.

NUTRITIONAL FACTS	
Serving Size	1 share
Calories	318 cal
Fats	24 g
Carbohydrates	4 g
Protein	23 g

Recipe #36 - Italian-Style Pan-Fried Broccoli

Servings: 2-4

Ingredients

- 2 cups Broccoli florets
- 6 Anchovies in olive oil
- 1 Long red chili, finely sliced
- 2-3 tbsp. Oil from the anchovies
- 2 tbsp. Pine nuts
- Pepper

Directions

1. Place a nonstick pan over medium heat and add the oil plus the red chili. Stir for about half a minute.

2. Add the anchovies and continue to stir until they start to break down.

3. Add the broccoli—still continuously stirring—until everything is mixed through.

4. Lower the heat and cover the pan with a lid. Let it cook for about 5-10 minutes or until the broccoli is tender. Don't hesitate to add a few tablespoons of water if needed.

5. Once the broccoli is okay, add the pines and season with pepper. Remove the pan from heat.

6. Transfer everything to a bowl and serve immediately.

NUTRITIONAL FACTS	
Serving Size	1 oz
Calories	4 cal
Fats	0.2 g
Carbohydrates	0.4 g
Protein	0.2 g

Recipe #37 - Smoked Salmon Breakfast Delight

Servings: 2

Ingredients

- 1 Hot-smoked salmon fillet, sugar-free and nitrate-free
- A handful Mixed salad leaves, washed
- 2 Free-range eggs
- 1 sprig Dill, chopped
- 2 tsp. Lemon juice
- ½ Lemon halved
- 2 tsp. Olive oil
- 1 tsp. Coconut oil

Directions

1. Whisk the eggs in a small bowl.

2. Place a nonstick pan over medium heat and melt the coconut oil. Pour the eggs and turn the pan to evenly cover the surface with it. Cook for a minute and flip. Continue to cook for another minute, so both sides become golden. Remove the omelet from the heat and let it cool down.

3. Once the omelet is cool enough to the touch, remove it from the pan. Roll it up like a crepe and cut into thin strips.

4. Next, put the salad leaves and dill into a bowl. Pour the olive oil and lemon juice over the salad.

5. Break the salmon fillet into flakes and add to the bowl. Add the omelet strips as well. Serve with a lemon wedge if desired.

NUTRITIONAL FACTS	
Serving Size	2 oz.
Calories	90 ca
Fats	1 g
Carbohydrates	2 g
Protein	11 g

Recipe #38 - Spicy Shrimp-Avocado Turret

Servings: 2

Ingredients

- 1 cup Cooked shrimp, peeled, tails removed and coarsely chopped
- 1 cup Avocado, diced
- 1 cup Cauliflower rice
- 1 cup Cucumber, peeled and diced
- 1 tbsp. Cilantro, finely chopped
- 1/3 cup Paleo mayonnaise
- 1 tbsp. Coconut Aminos
- 2 tsp. Sriracha sauce
- 1 tbsp. Sesame oil
- 1 tbsp. Sesame seeds
- Black pepper

Directions

1. To make the cauliflower rice, process the florets in a food processor until they're finely chopped.

2. Mix the cauliflower rice and sesame oil together and then set aside.

3. Mash the avocado in a small bowl until you achieve a moderately chunky consistency. Add the cilantro.

4. In a different bowl, mix in the shrimp and coconut aminos until the shrimp is thoroughly coated.

5. In another bowl, combine the mayonnaise with Sriracha sauce.

6. Using a one-cup measuring scoop, arrange the following in layers: ¼ cup cucumber, avocado, shrimp and cauliflower rice. Slightly press them into the cup to make a small turret.

7. Gently flip the measuring scoop on a plate. Release with a light tap on the bottom of the scoop. Do this to the remaining ingredients.

8. Garnish each turret with Sriracha-mayo mixture, sesame seeds, and pepper.

NUTRITIONAL FACTS	
Serving Size	1 cup
Calories	52.5 cal
Fats	1.1 g
Carbohydrates	9,1 g
Protein	1.3 g

Recipe #39 - Baked Sea Bass with Lemon Caper Dressing

Servings:

Ingredients

For the sea bass:

- 4 x 100g (or 4oz.) Sea bass fillets
- Olive oil, for brushing
- For the caper dressing:
- 2 tbsp. Small capers
- 2 tbsp. Flat-leaf parsley (plus a few extra leaves), chopped
- Zest from 1 lemon
- 2 tbsp. Lemon juice
- 2 tsp. Dijon mustard, gluten-free
- 3 tbsp. Extra virgin olive oil

Directions

1. For the dressing, combine the capers, lemon juice, zest, mustard, olive oil, and a tablespoon of water. Remember to leave out the parsley as the acid from the lemon would only fade its color. Put this only before serving.

2. Preheat the oven to 220°C.

3. Line a baking tray with parchment or foil. Place the fish with the skin-side up. Brush the skin with oil and season with salt. Cook for about 7 minutes or until the flesh of the bass becomes flaky when tested with a knife.

4. Once cooked, transfer fish to a plate. Top with dressing and parsley before serving.

NUTRITIONAL FACTS	
Serving Size	8 oz.
Calories	243 cal
Fats	5 g
Carbohydrates	12 g
Protein	1 g

Recipe #40 - Bacon Omelet Wedges - Summer Salad Recipe

Servings: 2-4

Ingredients

- 200g Smoked lardon
- 100g Brie, sliced
- 1 Cucumber, halved, deseeded and diagonally sliced
- 200g Radish quartered
- Small bunch chives, snipped
- 6 Eggs, lightly beaten
- 1 tsp. Dijon mustard
- 1 tsp. Red wine vinegar
- 2 tbsp. Olive oil
- Ground black pepper

Directions

1. Turn on the grill and heat a teaspoon of oil in a small pan. Place the lardons and cook until they're golden and crispy. Transfer to a plate lined with kitchen towel to drain excess oil.

2. Heat 2 tsp. of oil in a non-stick pan.

3. Combine the lardons, eggs, chives and ground black pepper. Pour the mixture into the pan and cook on low heat until the omelet is half-set. Place the brie on top and grill it until golden. Transfer the omelet to the plate and cut it into wedges.

4. Mix the mustard, vinegar, remaining oil, and seasoning in a large salad bowl. Add the radish and cucumber slices. Serve together with the omelet.

NUTRITIONAL FACTS	
Serving Size	1 Omelet
Calories	377 cal
Fats	30.7 g
Carbohydrates	7.1 g
Protein	7.3 g

Recipe #41 - Salmon and Spinach With Tartare Cream

Servings: 1-2

Ingredients

- 2 Skinless salmon fillets
- 250g bag Spinach
- 2 tbsp. Reduced-fat crème fraîche
- 1 tsp. Caper, drained
- 2 tbsp. Flat-leaf parsley, chopped
- Juice ½ lemon
- Lemon wedges
- 1 tsp. Olive oil

Directions

1. Place skillet over medium heat and pour the oil. Season the salmon on both sides and fry each side for

about 4 minutes or until golden and the flesh becomes flake when tested with a knife. Transfer to a plate and set aside.

2. Tip the spinach in the pan and season. Cover the pan with a lid and let the leaves wilt for about a minute, stirring them once halfway through. Divide the spinach between two plates and top with salmon.

3. Heat the crème Fraiche in a pan over low heat. Add the lemon juice, parsley, capers, and seasoning. Be careful not to let it boil. Pour sauce over fish and serve with lemon wedges.

NUTRITIONAL FACTS	
Serving Size	1 plate
Calories	321 cal
Fats	20 g
Carbohydrates	3 g
Protein	32 g

Recipe #42 - Quick and Easy Black Rice Mix

Servings: 2

Ingredients

- 100g Black rice
- 1L Water
- 8 Cherry tomatoes, quartered
- ½ Mild red chili, chopped
- ½ Red pepper
- 1 tbsp. Green spring onion leaves, chopped
- 1 tsp. Ginger, grated
- 2 tbsp. Fresh coriander, chopped
- ½ tsp. Caster sugar
- Juice of ½ lime
- 1 tbsp. Fish sauce

- 1 tbsp. Sesame oil

- Sea salt and black pepper

Directions

1. Put the rice in a saucepan with 1L water. Boil and let it simmer for a total of 25 minutes.

2. While you're boiling the rice, grill the pepper until the skin has charred. Let it cool for a bit before peeling off the skin. Cut into strips and set aside.

3. Drain the rice and transfer into a bowl. Add the pepper strips plus the remaining ingredients and mix the rice well. Serve and enjoy.

NUTRITIONAL FACTS	
Serving Size	Half cup
Calories	233 cal
Fats	5 g
Carbohydrates	39.9 g
Protein	7 g

Recipe #43 - Oat Porridge with Fruit Delight

Servings: 1

Ingredients

For the porridge:

- 23g Rolled oats or oat bran
- 150ml Water
- 2 tsp. Sunflower seeds
- 1 tsp. Vanilla sugar
- For serving:
- 80g Mixed fruits, chopped (blueberries, strawberries, raspberries, and clementines)
- 50ml Rice milk

Directions

1. Put oats and water in a saucepan and bring to a boil. Once it boils, reduce heat and let it simmer for a few

minutes. Remember to stir the porridge to bring out its creamy texture.

2. Meanwhile, dry-roast the seeds in a pan until they become golden.

3. Remove the saucepan containing the porridge from the stove. Mix in the seeds and milk.

4. Garnish the porridge with chopped fruits and vanilla sugar before serving.

NUTRITIONAL FACTS	
Serving Size	1 cup
Calories	199 cal
Fats	3.5
Carbohydrates	34.9
Protein	4.4

Recipe #44 - Coconut Chicken with Spinach

Servings: 2

Ingredients

- 2 cloves Garlic, finely sliced
- 2 Small chicken breasts
- 1 x 450 ml can Coconut milk
- 1 large bag Spinach leaves
- Olive oil

Directions

1. Place a small saucepan over medium heat and pour a small amount of olive oil. Once hot, cook the garlic for about half a minute or until it begins to turn brown.

2. Add the chicken and coconut milk, then bring to a simmer. Cook for another 5 minutes and cover with a lid.

3. Remove the saucepan from the heat and let it stand for 20 minutes.

4. Next, get the chicken and slice thinly. Divide between two serving plates.

5. Meanwhile, put the spinach into the saucepan and let it simmer until the leaves have wilted. Season if desired.

6. Top the chicken with the greens and pour the sauce over. Serve.

NUTRITIONAL FACTS	
Serving Size	9.8 oz
Calories	420 cal
Fats	10 g
Carbohydrates	36 g
Protein	44 g

Recipe #45 - Stir-Fried Gingered Salmon

Servings: 2

Ingredients

- 2 tbsp. Sesame oil
- 1 x 8oz. Wild salmon fillet, cut into large chunks
- 1 Organic carrot, cut into thin rounds
- 1 cup Snow peas, thinly sliced
- 1 bunch Scallions, diced
- 2 tbsp. Ginger, peeled and grated
- 1 garlic clove, peeled and minced
- ¼ cup Cashews (whole or pieces), dry-roasted
- Wheat-free tamari sauce
- Organic brown rice vinegar (or ume plum vinegar)

Directions

- Season the salmon chunks with salt and black pepper.

- Place a large skillet over high heat and pour the sesame oil. Once hot, cook the salmon chunks (2 minutes each side). After flipping the first time, immediately add the snow peas and carrots. When both sides are cooked, start to toss gently as you add garlic and ginger. Cook until the veggies are tender.

- Add a few splashes of vinegar and tamari, make adjustments if desired. Cover the pan with a lid and let it be for a minute or two. Toss a few times before serving.

NUTRITIONAL FACTS	
Serving Size	1 serve
Calories	304 cal
Fats	19.4 g
Carbohydrates	4.9 g
Protein	26 g

Recipe #46 - The Ultimate Healthy Gut Noodles

Servings: 2

Ingredients

- 1 Zucchini or Courgette
- 1 Ripe avocado
- 1 Carrot
- 1 cup of Peas
- A handful of Pumpkin Seeds
- A handful of Fresh Mint
- A large handful of Kale
- 1 tsp. of Olive oil
- 1 Lime or lemon
- Salt

Directions

1. Begin by boiling the peas. Use cold water for this step.

2. While boiling, make the carrot and zucchini (or courgette) noodles using a spiralizer.

3. Next, put the avocado, kale, mint, olive oil, and salt in a food processor. Pulse until you achieve a creamy consistency. Once the peas are cooked, add about ¾ of it and process again.

4. Combine pesto sauce with the noodles and garnish with pumpkin seeds.

NUTRITIONAL FACTS	
Serving Size	3 oz
Calories	20 cal
Fats	0 g
Carbohydrates	3 g
Protein	2 g

Recipe #47 - Kombucha

Serving: 2-4

Ingredients

- 6 Pcs. Green Tea bags

- 1.5 cups Unflavored Starter tea

- 1 SCOBY (Symbiotic Culture of Bacteria and Yeast)

Directions

1. Boil water in a stockpot. Remove from heat and add sugar. Add tea bags and leave the water to cool.

2. Once cooled, remove the tea bags and add the starter tea. This is important to acidify the mixture and prevent the formation of bacteria before the fermentation process.

3. Pour starter mixture into brewing jars and mix SCOBY using your hands. Make sure it is clean.

Secure paper towels over the top of the jar using an elastic band to cover.

4. From the 7th day, take a sample of the Kombucha to taste. If it tastes right, you can bottle it or pour into storage jars for storing in the fridge.

5. For added flavor, you may use herbs, fruits, or juice. Mix and let sit for 1-3 days at room temperature. If using bottle jars, make sure it is not getting too carbonated lest it will cause the bottle to explode. Store it in the fridge for up to 1 month.

NUTRITIONAL FACTS	
Serving Size	250 ml
Calories	30 cal
Fats	0 g
Carbohydrates	5 g
Protein	0 g

Recipe #48 - Crunchy Egg Roll

Serving: 1

Ingredients

Wrappers:

- 1/2 cup arrowroot starch
- 4 eggs
- 2 tbsp. coconut oil
- 1 tbsp. sesame oil
- 1/4 tsp. sea salt
- 3 tbsp. water

Filling:

- 1 cup Cabbage, shredded
- 1 tsp. Ginger, grated
- 2 tbsp. Sesame oil

- 1 cup Carrots, grated

- 2 tbsp. Green onions, chopped

- 1 clove Garlic, minced

- 1/2 cup Sliced mushrooms

- 2 tbsp. Coconut aminos

- 1/2 cup Broccoli, finely chopped

- 1/2 cup Red peppers, diced

- Ghee or lard, for frying

Directions

1. In making wrappers, combine all ingredients except the sesame oil and put these in a blender. Puree at the lowest speed.

2. Preheat a nonstick skillet over medium heat and pour sesame oil. Also, pour in the batter into the pan to form a 4-inch circle. Cook for about a minute and

then flip to cook the other side. Transfer to a platter and continue cooking the remaining mixture for additional wrappers. Let cool while preparing for the filling.

3. To do the filling, heat sesame oil in a large skillet. Saute the green onions, garlic, and ginger. Add remaining ingredients and cook until soft while continuously stirring. Remove from heat and allow to cool.

4. Heat the skillet and then add enough fat.

5. Meanwhile, lay wrappers on a flat surface and then place a spoonful of the filling in the middle. Carefully wrap around the mixture before putting it in the hot skillet. Using tongs, hold it rigidly until wrapper is set before releasing it completely. Carefully turn it until equally brown on all sides then transfer it to a paper towel-lined platter.

NUTRITIONAL FACTS	
Serving Size	1 serve
Calories	190 cal
Fats	7 g
Carbohydrates	25 g
Protein	3 g

Recipe #49 - Daikon-Endive Salad

Serving:

Ingredients

For Salad:

- 2 Endives, chopped
- 4 cups Daikon, peeled and freshly grated
- 2 Carrots, peeled and grated
- 2 tbsp. Fresh mint, chopped
- 1tsp. Rice malt syrup
- juice of 1 lemon
- 2 tbsp. Fresh coriander, chopped
- ½ tsp. Celtic Sea salt

For Dressing:

- 1/2 tsp. Minced ginger

- ½ cup Tahini

- 2 tbsps. Rice malt syrup

- zest of one lemon

- ½ tsp. Cinnamon

- ½ tsp. Ground turmeric

- 1 tsp. Ground coriander

- 1 tsp. Ground cumin

- A pinch of cayenne pepper

- 1 cup Coconut milk or homemade 24-hour yogurt

- 2 tbsps. Cider vinegar

- juice of 1 lemon

- Hazelnuts (crushed), fresh coriander, and fresh mint to garnish

Directions

- Mix daikon, endive, and carrots in a mixing bowl. Toss to blend.

- In a separate large mixing bowl, combine lemon, rice malt syrup, coriander, mint, and salt. Whisk together.

- Mix all together with daikon, endive, and carrots and marinate for about 15-30 minutes.

- In another bowl, prepare the dressing by mixing the coconut milk or 24-hour homemade yogurt, lemon juice and zest, tahini, rice malt syrup, and apple cider vinegar. Also add the coriander, cumin, turmeric, ginger, cayenne pepper, and cinnamon. Mix well to blend and store in the refrigerator to chill.

- Serve with crushed hazelnut, mint, and coriander.

NUTRITIONAL FACTS	
Serving Size	100 gram
Calories	17 cal
Fats	0.2 g
Carbohydrates	3.4 g
Protein	1.3 g

Recipe #50 - Zucchini Pasta with Sausage and Roasted Garlic Sauce

Serving: 1

Ingredients

- 2 Small zucchini, cut into pasta
- 2 tbsp. Roasted garlic
- 2 tbsp. Olive oil
- 1/4 cup Additive-free Coconut Milk or Homemade 24-hour yogurt
- 2 Pcs, All natural, sugar-free Sausage, fully cooked
- Salt, to taste

Directions

1. Prepare a small pot of water and bring to boil. Add zucchini pasta to the boiling water and cook for about a minute to soften. Remove from heat and discard water to drain.

2. In a separate small saute pan, heat olive oil over medium heat. Remove sausage casing, though it naturally peels off once sausage becomes cold. Slice the sausages and cook in olive oil until these turn brown. Remove from pan and set aside to cool.

3. With the remaining olive oil in the pan, add roasted garlic and coconut milk. Warm it over low fire and season the season the sauce with salt to taste.

4. Prepare pasta and sausages in a platter and top it with the warm sauce. Enjoy!

NUTRITIONAL FACTS	
Serving Size	4 oz
Calories	220 cal
Fats	20 g
Carbohydrates	5 g
Protein	11 g

Final Words

Thank you again for purchasing this book! I really hope this book is able to help you.

The next step is for you to **join our email newsletter** to receive updates on any upcoming new book releases or promotions. You can sign-up for free and as a bonus, you will also receive our "*7 Fitness Mistakes You Don't Know You're Making*" book! This bonus book breaks down many of the most common fitness mistakes and will demystify many of the complexities and science of getting into shape. Having all this fitness knowledge and science organized into an actionable step-by-step book will help you get started in the right direction in your fitness journey! To join our free email newsletter and grab your free book, please visit the link and signup: **www.hmwpublishing.com/gift**

Finally, if you enjoyed this book, then I would like to ask you for a favor, would you be kind enough to leave a review for this book? It would be greatly appreciated!

Thank you and good luck in your journey!

About the Co-Author

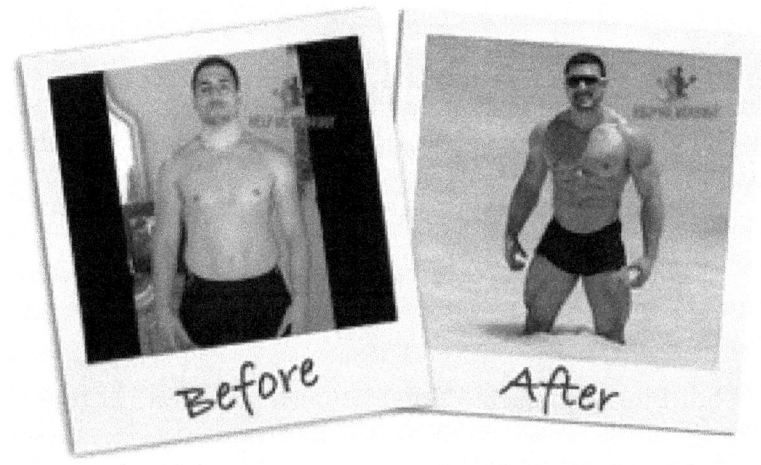

My name is George Kaplo; I'm a certified personal trainer from Montreal, Canada. I'll start off by saying I'm not the biggest guy you will ever meet and this has never really been my goal. In fact, I started working out to overcome my biggest insecurity when I was younger, which was my self-confidence. This was due to my height measuring only 5 foot 5 inches (168cm), it pushed me down to attempt anything I ever wanted to achieve in life. You may be going through some challenges right now, or you may simply want to get fit, and I can certainly relate.

For me personally, I was always kind of interested in the health & fitness world and wanted to gain some muscle due to the numerous bullying in my teenage years about my height and my overweight body. I figured I couldn't do anything about my height, but I sure can do something about how my body looked like. This was the beginning of my transformation journey. I had no idea where to start, but I just got started. I felt worried and afraid at times that other people would make fun of me for doing the exercises the wrong way. I always wished I had a friend that was next to me who was knowledgeable enough to help me get started and "show me the ropes."

After a lot of work, studying and countless trial and errors. Some people began to notice how I was getting more fit and how I was starting to form a keen interest in the topic. This led many friends and new faces to come to me and ask me for fitness advice. At first, it seemed odd when people asked me to help them get in shape. But what kept me going is when they started to see changes in their own body and told me it's the first time that they saw real results!

From there, more people kept coming to me, and it made me realize after so much reading and studying in this field that it did help me but it also allowed me to help others. I'm now a fully certified personal trainer and have trained numerous clients to date who have achieved amazing results.

Today, my brother Alex Kaplo (also a Certified Personal Trainer) and I own & operate this publishing venture, where we bring passionate and expert authors to write about health and fitness topics. We also run an online fitness website "HelpMeWorkout.com" and I would love to connect with by inviting you to visit the website on the following page and signing up to our e-mail newsletter (you will even get a free book).

Last but not least, if you are in the position I was once in and you want some guidance, don't hesitate and ask... I'll be there to help you out!

Your friend and coach,

George Kaplo
Certified Personal Trainer

Get another book for Free

I want to thank you for purchasing this book and offer you another book (just as long and valuable as this book), "Health & Fitness Mistakes You Don't Know You're Making", completely free.

Visit the link below to signup and receive it:

www.hmwpublishing.com/gift

In this book, I will break down the most common health & fitness mistakes, you are probably committing right now, and I will reveal how you can easily get in the best shape of your life!

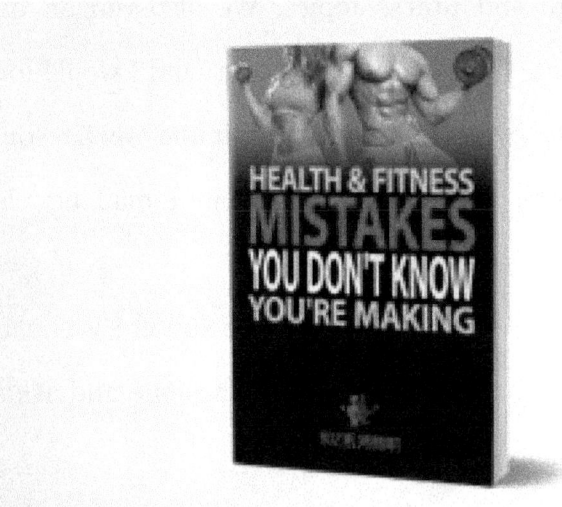

In addition to this valuable gift, you will also have an opportunity to get our new books for free, enter giveaways, and receive other valuable emails from me. Again, visit the link to sign up:

www.hmwpublishing.com/gift

Copyright 2017 by HMW Publishing - All Rights Reserved.

This document by HMW Publishing owned by the A&G Direct Inc company, is geared towards providing exact and reliable information in regards to the topic and issue covered. The publication is sold with the idea that the publisher is not required to render accounting, officially permitted, or otherwise, qualified services. If advice is necessary, legal or professional, a practiced individual in the profession should be ordered.

From a Declaration of Principles which was accepted and approved equally by a Committee of the American Bar Association and a Committee of Publishers and Associations.

In no way is it legal to reproduce, duplicate, or transmit any part of this document in either electronic means or in printed format. Recording of this publication is strictly prohibited, and any storage of this document is not allowed unless with written permission from the publisher. All rights reserved.

The information provided herein is stated to be truthful and consistent, in that any liability, in terms of inattention or otherwise, by any usage or abuse of any policies, processes, or directions contained within is the solitary and utter responsibility of the recipient reader. Under no circumstances will any legal responsibility or blame be held against the publisher for any reparation, damages, or monetary loss due to the information herein, either directly or indirectly.

The information herein is offered for informational purposes solely, and is universal as so. The presentation of the information is without contract or any type of guarantee assurance.

The trademarks that are used are without any consent, and the publication of the trademark is without permission or backing by the trademark owner. All trademarks and brands within this book are for clarifying purposes only and are the owned by the owners themselves, not affiliated with this document.

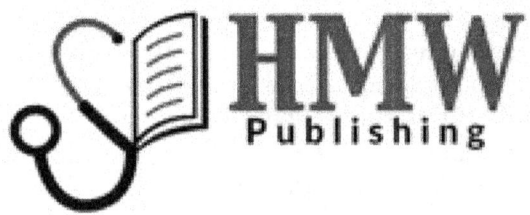

For more great books visit:

HMWPublishing.com

www.ingramcontent.com/pod-product-compliance
Lightning Source LLC
Chambersburg PA
CBHW070029040426
42333CB00040B/1255